CRITERIA FOR NURSING EXCELLENCE

TRANSFORMATIONAL
LEADERSHIP

ANCC
AMERICAN NURSES CREDENTIALING CENTER
MAGNET

Visit www.nursecredentialing.org/magnet for manual updates.

AMERICAN NURSES CREDENTIALING CENTER

The American Nurses Credentialing Center (ANCC) provides people and organizations in the nursing profession with the tools they need on their journey to excellence. ANCC recognizes healthcare organizations for nursing excellence through the Magnet Recognition Program®. ANCC is the largest and most prestigious nurse-credentialing organization in the United States.

Commission on Magnet® Recognition

The ANCC's Commission on Magnet® Recognition is a voluntary governing body that oversees the Magnet Recognition Program. Commission members are appointed by the ANCC's board of directors and are representatives from various sectors of the nursing community, which includes nursing executive leaders, nurse managers, staff nurses, long-term-care nurses, and advanced practice registered nurses. One commission member represents public consumers. The Commission on Magnet Recognition makes the final determination of award designation.

Magnet® Appraisers

Appraisers are leading expert nurses with demonstrated expertise and experience in various organizational and specialty backgrounds relevant to the Magnet Recognition Program. They evaluate applicant documents, conduct site visits, and prepare the final report to the Commission on Magnet Recognition. Appraisers are selected through a competitive application process. All appraisers undergo intensive training on the interpretation and evaluation of Sources of Evidence for the Magnet appraisal process before being assigned to any appraiser team.

Magnet® Program Office

The ANCC's Magnet program office staff manages and coordinates all aspects of the application and appraisal process. Contact information is available at www.nursecredentialing.org/magnet/magnetcontacts.

Published by American Nurses Credentialing Center
8515 Georgia Avenue, Suite 400
Silver Spring, MD 20910-3492

Copyright ©2017 by American Nurses Credentialing Center, Silver Spring, MD
2019 edition. A subsidiary of the American Nurses Association

ISBN print: 978-1-947800-04-5
ISBN epdf: 978-1-947800-03-8
ISBN ePub: 978-1-947800-05-2
ISBN mobi: 978-1-947800-06-9

Disclaimers:

Please note: this is an abridged version of the Magnet Recognition Program Application Manual. If your organization is considering pursuing Magnet recognition, the 2019 edition of the Magnet Manual is essential for understanding the full scope of application requirements. It is the only authorized publication that provides detailed information on the instructions and process for documentation submission. To order a copy of the 2019 Magnet Manual or obtain additional information about the Magnet Recognition Program, visit our website at www.nursecredentialing.org/magnet.

The Magnet Vision

Magnet® organizations will serve as the fount of knowledge and expertise for the delivery of nursing care globally. They will be solidly grounded in core Magnet principles, flexible, and constantly striving for discovery and innovation. They will lead the reformation of health care; the discipline of nursing; and care of the patient, family, and community.

—*The Commission on Magnet Recognition, 2008*

Contents

THE MAGNET VISION   III

PREFACE   VII

CHAPTER 1   THE MAGNET® MODEL.....................1
Statistical Foundation: The Empirical Model   2

CHAPTER 2   ORGANIZATIONAL OVERVIEW AND SOURCES OF EVIDENCE: NARRATIVE AND DOCUMENTATION REQUIREMENTS 5
Organizational Overview   5
Source of Evidence (SOE) Example Types   6

SECTION II   TRANSFORMATIONAL LEADERSHIP (TL) 9
Organizational Overview   10
Empirical Outcomes   11
Sources of Evidence (SOEs)   15
Compliance with Local, State, and Federal Laws and Regulations   19
Preparation of Written Documentation   21

APPENDIX A   MAGNET RECOGNITION PROGRAM® RESOURCES 23
Magnet Recognition Program Staff   23
The Magnet Recognition Program Website   25
Critical Information Webinar   26
In Pursuit of Excellence: Magnet Recognition Program® Guidance   26
Annual ANCC National Magnet Conference®   26

KEY TERMS   29

REFERENCES   39

Preface

On behalf of the American Nurses Credentialing Center (ANCC), we are pleased to present the 2019 edition of ANCC's *Magnet® Application Manual*. This valuable resource contains information and instructions to guide Magnet-recognized organizations and those considering the Journey to Magnet Excellence™.

ANCC's Magnet designation is the highest and most prestigious credential a healthcare organization can achieve for nursing excellence and quality patient care. This outcomes-driven credential brings both external prestige and wide-ranging internal benefits including improved patient outcomes, nurse satisfaction and retention, and reduced costs.

The revisions to the 2019 *Magnet® Application Manual* are rooted in a strong evidence base which spans twenty years of research and development. They create relevance for the Magnet journey by relating to the significant changes we are seeing in healthcare delivery systems around the world. The 2019 Manual clarifies previous standards, reduces the amount of information requested, and further simplifies the document submission process. Our continued focus on and strengthening of the outcomes standards will help all organizations demonstrate the value nursing brings to the patient, the organization, and the community.

Magnet designation is available to any healthcare organization regardless of size, setting, or location. Many organizations find the Journey to Magnet Excellence a valuable process to identify and improve processes, nursing structure, and ultimately deliver stronger, patient-centered outcomes.

The 2019 standards continue to raise the bar as the gold standard for nursing care delivery, new nursing knowledge, and evidence-based clinical quality in healthcare organizations around the world. The Commission on Magnet Recognition and ANCC's Magnet Recognition Program® staff trust that the 2019 *Magnet® Application Manual* will strengthen your commitment to these values and inspire you on the Journey to Magnet Excellence.

Donna S. Havens, PhD, RN, FAAN
Chair, Commission on Magnet Recognition

Jeffrey N. Doucette, DNP, RN, CENP, FACHE, NEA-BC
Vice President, Magnet Recognition Program

THE MAGNET® MODEL

The Forces of Magnetism that were identified more than thirty years ago have remained remarkably stable—a testament to their enduring value. The Magnet Recognition Program® evolved over time in response to changes in the healthcare environment.

Figure 1.1. Triaxial Diagram

Statistical Foundation: The Empirical Model

In 2007, the American Nurses Credentialing Center (ANCC) commissioned a statistical analysis of final appraisal scores for applicants under the 2005 *Magnet Recognition Program Application Manual* (ANCC 2004). The project goal was to examine the relationships among the Forces of Magnetism by investigating alternative frameworks for structuring the **Sources of Evidence**[*] (SOEs)

---

[*] This formatting indicates that these words and phrases are defined in the Key Terms. Please refer to the Key Terms on pages 29–37 for full explanations of these terms.

and to inform development of the new Magnet Model. The newly developed Magnet Model provided a new perspective on the SOEs and how they interplay to create a work environment that supports excellence in nursing.

Through a combination of factor analysis, cluster analysis, and multidimensional scaling, the final SOEs scores were examined to determine how they might be organized based solely on their empirical properties. The results suggested an alternative framework for grouping the SOEs. The empiric model yielded from this analysis informed the conceptual development of the current Magnet Model.

Each subsequent manual has utilized a similar rigorous process, resulting in Magnet organizations creating a continued culture of excellence and innovation in nursing. Excellence is determined through the evaluation of examples demonstrating the infrastructure for excellence. The examples, provided by Magnet organizations, incorporate the structure and process used to achieve improved outcomes demonstrate how the structures and processes are present and operationalized within the organization.

Any narrative addressing SOEs must reflect compliance across the breadth and depth of the organization, wherever nursing is practiced. The Magnet program office (MPO) conducted an extensive review of final appraisal reports for written documentation that supported a site visit and incorporated the results into the 2019 Application Manual. Successful organizations demonstrated the development, dissemination, and enculturation of the Sources of Evidence.

Chapter 2

ORGANIZATIONAL OVERVIEW AND SOURCES OF EVIDENCE: NARRATIVE AND DOCUMENTATION REQUIREMENTS

Organizational Overview

The Organizational Overview requests documents and information that are foundational to Magnet® Organizations. In order for the appraisers to progress to the review of the component Sources of Evidence (SOEs), verification of all Organizational Overview items must first occur. If it is determined that any Organizational Overview items are missing, the applicant will be given the opportunity to provide the missing information one time only. If this should occur, the evaluation of the healthcare organization's documentation for Magnet designation under the Magnet Recognition Program® will be temporarily suspended and the evaluation process will not proceed until the requested information has been received. Organizations will have five business days to provide the requested information. After receipt of the organization overview items, the review will resume. When this review is concluded, the possible outcomes are a site visit, request for additional documentation, or denial.

Source of Evidence (SOE) Example Types

It is important to understand the SOE types before writing to the requirement. The SOE type will determine the format and **supporting evidence** required.

The 2019 Magnet® Application Manual contains two types of SOE examples:

EMPIRICAL OUTCOMES (EOS)

▸ Follow presentation guidelines found on page 11.

▸ Evidence must be presented as outcome data.

▸ All data must be within the forty-eight-month timeline.

▸ A limited number of EO sources require specific supporting documentation.

▸ Unique EO presentations are required for nurse **certification**, nurse education, **nurse satisfaction**, nurse-sensitive indicators, and **patient satisfaction**. Presentation requirements can be found with the corresponding SOE.

SOURCES OF EVIDENCE (SOES) NOT INCLUDING EMPIRICAL OUTCOMES (EOS)

Applicants will write narrative statements to address the SOEs. Descriptions of processes or programs must be accompanied by examples to illustrate how each is operationalized. The written document should provide examples from different departments or units to represent a variety of specialties and nursing leadership.

The applicant is required to submit a separate narrative for each SOE.

The applicant must clearly identify the SOE being addressed in each piece of the narrative.

▸ Narrative statements should be straightforward and concise and should not include extraneous information.

▸ Evidence should support and substantiate the narrative, providing verification that what is stated in the narrative actually exists in the organization.

▸ Evidence is limited to five items per SOE example.

Note: Examples of acceptable evidence include copies of policies and procedures, meeting minutes, various types of correspondence, data, rosters, and screenshots. Photographs and testimonials are not considered evidence.

TRANSFORMATIONAL LEADERSHIP (TL)

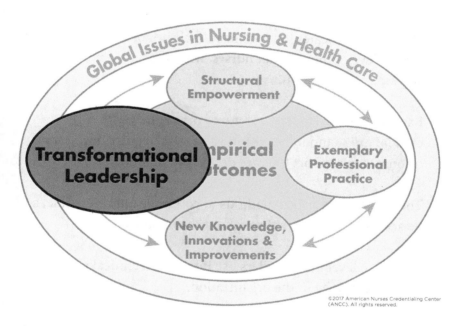

The intent of the **Transformational Leadership*** component is to reflect:

▸ Nursing's **mission**, **vision**, values, and strategic plan align with the organization's priorities to improve the organization's performance.

---

* This formatting indicates that these words and phrases are defined in the Key Terms. Please refer to the Key Terms on pages 29–37 for full explanations of these terms.

- Nurses advocate for resources to support nursing unit and organizational goals.

- The CNO influences organization-wide change beyond the scope of nursing.

- The CNO is a strategic partner in the organization's decision-making.

- Nurse leaders lead effectively through change.

- The CNO advocates for organizational support of ongoing leadership development for all nurses, with a focus on mentoring and succession planning.

- Executive nurse leaders and nurse managers, with clinical nurse input, use trended data to acquire necessary resources to support the care delivery system(s).

- The CNO uses various methods to communicate, be visible, and be accessible to nurses throughout the organization.

- Executive level nurse leaders use input from clinical nurses to influence change in the organization.

Organizational Overview

Organizational Overview documents provide information that are foundational for the structures and processes enculturated in a Magnet organization. The following Organizational Overview items are associated with the Sources of Evidence in the Transformational Leadership Component.

TRANSFORMATIONAL LEADERSHIP

1. Provide:

   ▸ The current chief nursing officer's (CNO) job description

   ▸ CNO's curriculum vitae or résumé

   ▸ The organizational chart(s)

   ▸ The nursing organizational chart(s)

   ▸ A description of the CNO's structural and operational relationships to all areas in which nursing is practiced

   ▸ Names and credentials, of all individuals serving as the CNO, in the forty-eight months preceding document submission. Include the tenure dates.

Empirical Outcomes

Throughout this application manual, in each of the model components, the EOs are requested as SOEs.

For all Transformational Leadership Empirical Outcomes presentations, follow the directions below.

When responding to an EO, both the goal statement and the supporting evidence must address an outcome measure. The data is best presented as a ratio (e.g., rates, percentiles, percentages). There are limited exceptions for raw data, such as **sentinel event** data.

Narratives must be presented using the following format:

Problem

▸ Describe the problem that you worked to improve

▸ Describe the pre-intervention outcome data that drove the goal and initiative (must have occurred within the forty-eight months prior to documentation submission)

Goal statement

▸ State the goal(s) that is the desired improvement

▸ Identify the outcome measure that aligns with the goal to demonstrate the improvement(s) (e.g., **errors**, incidents, satisfaction, clinical indicator)

▸ Include the location of the desired improvement

Participants

▸ List participants involved in the planning and intervention or initiative. Include name, discipline, title, and department.

Description of the intervention

▸ Activities that took place to facilitate change or improvement (include the dates of the work).

▸ Describe the action(s) that had an impact on the problem and resulted in the achievement of the outcome.

▶ Include where the intervention(s) occurred (e.g., unit, department, product line, organization).

▶ Include the timeline of date(s) when the intervention(s) or initiative(s) took place.

▶ The pre-intervention data and interventions) must have occurred within the forty-eight months prior to documentation submission.

Outcome

▶ For Magnet purposes, an outcome is quantitative evidence related to the impact of structure and process (intervention) on the patient, nursing workforce, organization, and consumer. These outcomes are dynamic and measurable.

▶ Trended data (minimum of one pre-intervention data point and three post-intervention data points) demonstrating an improved trend.

▶ Pre-intervention data and post-intervention data must be displayed to indicate the effect of an intervention.

▶ The trended data must be displayed as a graph and table with data elements clearly provided.

Data display requirements

▶ The graph must include dates, times, location of intervention, and title.

▶ A legend must be included.

▸ Indicate on the graph the date(s) for pre-intervention data, intervention(s) or initiative(s), and post-intervention data.

▸ The x-axis units-of-time must be the same for pre-intervention, intervention, and post-intervention data (e.g., quarters, months).

▸ The y-axis units of measure represent the desired outcome. Data must be presented as ratio (e.g., rates, percentiles, percentages). Additionally, the unit of measure (e.g., percent to percent, whole number to whole number) must be consistent throughout the data collection period.

▸ If data are presented for a fiscal year, the period of time defining the fiscal year must be defined with calendar year equivalent (January to December and year; June to May and year).

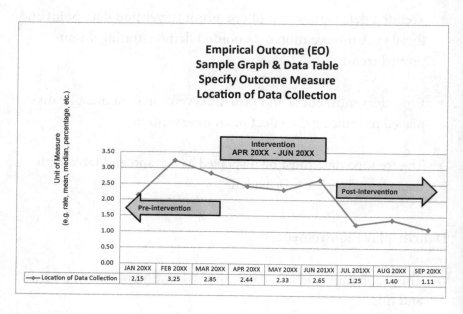

Figure II.1 Empirical Outcomes (EO) Sample Graph and Data Table

Sources of Evidence (SOEs)

Source of Evidence (excluding Empirical Outcomes)

▸ Each key element within the SOE must be described and supported with evidence.

▸ Limit evidence to no more than five items per SOE example.

▸ Ensure all protected health information (PHI) has been redacted.

Note: All organizations with **ambulatory care setting(s)** are required to provide a minimum of one ambulatory care example for TL6 and TL7.

STRATEGIC PLANNING

TL1:

a. Provide one example, with supporting evidence, of an initiative in nursing practice that is consistent with the organization's mission statement.

▸ Provide a copy of the organization's mission statement as one of the supporting documents.

TL2EO:

a. Provide one example, with supporting evidence, of an improved patient outcome associated with a goal in the nursing strategic plan.

- Patient outcome data must be submitted in the form of a graph with a data table.
- Provide a copy of the nursing strategic plan.

ADVOCACY AND INFLUENCE

TL3:

a. Provide one example, with supporting evidence, of an **assistant vice president's** (AVP's)/nurse **director's** advocacy for resources to support an organizational goal.

  AND

a. Provide one example, with supporting evidence, of a nurse managers' advocacy for resources to support a unit goal.

TL4:

a. Provide one example, with supporting evidence, of the CNO's leadership that led to a strategic organizational change.

Note: Organizational change must be inclusive of nursing and other departments.

TL5EO:

a. Provide one example, with supporting evidence, of an improved patient outcome, associated with an AVP's/nurse director's, or nurse manager's membership in an organization-level, decision-making group.

- Patient outcome data may be presented at the organizational, division, or unit-level.

- Outcome data must be submitted in the form of a graph with a data table.

TL6:

Choose three of the following (**one example *must* be from** ambulatory care setting, **if applicable**):

a. Provide one example, with supporting evidence, of a mentoring plan or program for clinical nurse(s).

b. Provide one example, with supporting evidence, of a mentoring plan or program for nurse managers.

c. Provide one example, with supporting evidence, of a mentoring plan or program for AVPs/nurse directors (exclusive of nurse managers).

d. Provide one example, with supporting evidence, of a mentoring plan or program for **advanced practice registered nurses** (APRNs).

e. Provide one example, with supporting evidence, of a mentoring plan or program for the CNO.

TL7:

Choose three of the following (**one example *must* be from ambulatory care setting, if applicable**):

a. Provide one example, with supporting evidence, of succession-planning activities for the nurse manager role.

b. Provide one example, with supporting evidence, of succession-planning activities for the APRN role.

c. Provide one example, with supporting evidence, of succession-planning activities for the AVP/nurse director role.

d. Provide one example, with supporting evidence, of succession-planning activities for the CNO role.

TL8:

a. Provide one example, with supporting evidence, where a clinical nurse(s) utilized data to advocate for the acquisition of a resource, in support of the care delivery system(s).

VISIBILITY, ACCESSIBILITY, AND COMMUNICATION

TL9EO:

Choose two of the following:

a. Provide one example, with supporting evidence, of an improvement in patient care or the **nursing practice environment**, associated with communication between the clinical nurse(s) and the CNO.

▶ Outcome data must be submitted in the form of a graph with a data table.

b. Provide one example, with supporting evidence, of an improvement in patient care or the nursing practice environment, associated with communication between the clinical nurse(s) and the AVP/nurse director.

▶ Outcome data must be submitted in the form of a graph with a data table.

c. Provide one example, with supporting evidence, of an improvement in patient care or the nurse practice environment, associated, with communication between the clinical nurse(s) and a nurse manager.

▶ Outcome data must be submitted in the form of a graph with a data table.

Compliance with Local, State, and Federal Laws and Regulations

CONFIDENTIAL INFORMATION

In accordance with the Health Insurance Portability and Accountability Act (HIPAA) and other laws and regulations, inclusion of patient-specific information and employee-specific information as exhibits must be avoided. The original document should then be available for review during the site visit. Where state law prohibits review of a document, it would be exempt from display in the organization.

Applicant entities must comply with all local, state, and federal laws and regulations administered by the Occupational Safety and

Health Review Commission; the Equal Employment Opportunity Commission; the US Department of Health and Human Services and other agencies that administer healthcare programs; and the US Department of Labor, the **National Labor Relations Board** (NLRB), or other agencies as they relate to **registered nurses** in the workplace. Conduct by an applicant or a Magnet®-recognized organization that results in an adverse decision by the NLRB on an unfair labor practice **complaint** (adoption or modification of a decision rendered by an administrative law judge); a trial court decision on a complaint of employment discrimination; a decision by the Occupational Safety and Health Administration (OSHA) regarding violations of health and **safety** requirements; or the suspension or exclusion of a hospital from participation in a federal healthcare program will warrant review and action by the Commission on Magnet Recognition (COM).

Note: If protected health information (PHI) is found during the review process, the organization will be notified and be given a deadline to remove from all sources. The appraisers will stop the review if patient-sensitive information is identified.

All identified PHI must be removed. The appraisers will provide the Sources of Evidence (SOEs) where PHI has been identified. There may be other areas in the documentation that contain PHI and it is the responsibility of the organization to find and remove or redact this information. The organization's privacy officer must be notified if PHI is identified in the written documentation. If the revised documents are not provided within the required timeline, the review is concluded.

Applicant and Magnet-recognized healthcare organizations are required to disclose, within seven business days after receipt of such a decision, all decisions by an agency or court of law that occurred within the year before application or at any time after an application is submitted. Failure of an applicant or Magnet-recognized health-care organizations to report an adverse decision by the NLRB on an unfair labor practice complaint (adoption or modification of a decision rendered by an administrative law judge); a trial court decision on a complaint of employment discrimination; a decision by OSHA regarding violations of health and safety requirements; or the suspension or exclusion of a hospital from participation in a federal healthcare program may result in denial of a pending application for initial designation or redesignation, revocation of recognition, or other adverse action.

Organizations that have their Magnet designation revoked or are prevented from continuing the application process because of an adverse decision are prohibited from reapplying for Magnet designation for a period of one year after the adverse decision.

Preparation of Written Documentation

The required contents submitted for review contributes information critical to the appraisal process. This content includes:

▸ Demographic report submitted via the DDCT portal

▸ Organizational overview

▸ SOEs

Timeline:

▸ All narrative and evidence must occur within the forty-eight months prior to document submission. This includes narratives, data, and supporting evidence and exhibits.

- Nurse satisfaction must be within thirty months prior to document submission.

- Nurse-sensitive indicators (inpatient and ambulatory) and patient satisfaction (inpatient and ambulatory) must be the most recent eight quarters.

The SOEs statements in the 2019 Magnet® Application Manual depict requirements that are present and fully operational in Magnet-recognized healthcare organizations. The term Source of Evidence should not be confused with the reference to "evidence" that is required substantiating the narrative for the example.

Appendix A

MAGNET RECOGNITION PROGRAM® RESOURCES

Magnet Recognition Program Staff

SENIOR MAGNET® PROGRAM ANALYSTS (SMPA)

Nurses who provide independent content expertise and analysis for the Magnet Recognition Program, working with applicants, commissioners, appraisers, Magnet organizations, Magnet Program staff, and American Nurses Credentialing Center (ANCC) staff. They interface with Magnet appraisers to coordinate and manage the appraisal process and with representatives of the international community to provide guidance and interpretative analysis related to eligibility and requirements for Magnet Recognition®.

SENIOR MAGNET PROGRAM OUTCOMES ANALYST

Senior Magnet program outcomes analyst provides operational support and coordination to organizations between Magnet designations. Oversees the Demographic Data Collection Tool™ (DDCT), a web-based portal for managing compilation of required demographic data into a report. Interfaces with staff of Magnet-recognized organizations and those seeking the Magnet credential.

MAGNET PROGRAM SPECIALISTS (MPS)

Magnet program specialists (MPS) provide logistical support for the Magnet Recognition Program. Coordinate and monitor the activities of applicant and Magnet-recognized organizations throughout the various stages of the Magnet application process. Specialists interface with senior Magnet program analysts on a routine basis to ensure excellence and quality service throughout the Magnet application process.

SENIOR OPERATIONS SPECIALIST

Senior operations specialist provides operational and logistical support to the Magnet Program Staff with a variety of Magnet programs and presentations. Assists with conducting ongoing evaluation of Magnet Recognition Program processes for the Commission on Magnet Recognition(COM), appraiser pool, staff, and Magnet Recognition Program to ensure efficiency, effectiveness, and excellent customer service.

MAGNET RECOGNITION PROGRAM LEADERSHIP

Vice President, Magnet Recognition Program and Pathway to Excellence®

Director, Magnet Recognition Program

Senior Manager, Operations Magnet Recognition Program

Senior Manager, Magnet Appraiser Program

The Magnet Recognition Program Website

http://nursecredentialing.org/Magnet:

▶ Application

▶ Manual updates

▶ Frequently asked questions (FAQs)

▶ Forms and Templates (for example, unit-level crosswalk, nurse leader and nurse manager tables, nursing research table, template for internal review board attestation)

MAGNET LEARNING COMMUNITIES® (MLC) SUBSCRIPTION

▶ Two free memberships are provided with designation

▶ Applicants and those on the journey may purchase a membership; fees for subscription are located on our website: http://www.nursecredentialing.org/Magnet/Magnet-Learning/About.

The MLC provides the following:

▶ Discussion Forums: The forums include moderated discussions that bring together nurse leaders who share knowledge and experiences related to leadership, engagement, evidence-based practice, research, innovation, and outcomes.

▶ Education: Resources available on demand in the MLC, including the "Getting Started" webinar (provides an overview of resources, definitions, and formatting), educational vignettes (webinars lasting less than ten minutes), and more!

Critical Information Webinar

This is an invitation-only webinar, limited to Magnet and applicant organizations. The invitation is sent to the applicant chief nursing officer (CNO) and Magnet program director (MPD) when the Magnet application is received by the Magnet Program Office (MPO). Check with your assigned SMPA or MPS for registration.

In Pursuit of Excellence: Magnet Recognition Program® Guidance

This interactive work session is provided to expand the understanding of the requirements in the Magnet Application Manual. Required key elements of the organizational overview and Sources of Evidence (SOE) examples, as well as expectations for Empirical Outcome (EO) SOE data presentation, are reviewed in depth. Senior analysts present sample SOE examples, facilitate group discussion, and provide one-on-one assistance to enhance the attendees' understanding of SOEs while developing skills to successfully write to the Magnet requirements.

The class is limited to CNOs, MPDs, and key stakeholders from Magnetrecognized and Magnet applicant organizations.

Annual ANCC National Magnet Conference®

PRECONFERENCE

▸ In Pursuit of Excellence: Magnet Recognition Program Guidance

- Annual MPD session:

  - For MPDs of Magnet-recognized and Magnet applicant organizations.

DURING THE CONFERENCE

- Concurrent sessions are offered by the senior magnet program analysts.

- In addition, the senior Magnet program analysts are available for questions at the Magnet Recognition Program booth throughout the conference.

Key Terms

For full glossary of terms see 2019 Magnet Application Manual Glossary

advanced practice registered nurse (APRN)

A registered nurse who has met advanced educational and clinical practice requirements beyond the two to four years of basic nursing education required of all RNs. Under this umbrella are four principal types of APRNs: nurse practitioners, certified nurse midwives, clinical nurse specialists, and certified registered nurse anesthetists.

ambulatory care setting

"Ambulatory care nursing occurs across the continuum of care in a variety of settings, which include but are not limited to hospital-based clinic/centers, solo or group medical practices, ambulatory surgery, and diagnostic procedure centers, telehealth service environments, university and community hospital clinics, military and veterans administration settings, nurse-managed clinics, managed care organizations, colleges and educational institutions, free standing community facilities, care coordination organizations, and patient homes" (American Academy of Ambulatory Care Nursing 2011, 4). For Magnet® purposes, ambulatory care settings include emergency departments and emergency care.

assistant vice president (AVP)

Nurses with line authority over multiple units that have RNs working who deliver nursing care in an inpatient or ambulatory care setting and are positioned on the organizational chart between the nurse manager and the chief nursing officer. This may include registered nurses who may broadly influence or impact the clinical practice of nurses in the organization. If these nurses are referenced as an AVP in the organization's Magnet® application, they must meet the educational criteria (bachelor's in nursing or higher) and report directly or indirectly to the CNO. Examples may include AVPs responsible for, but are not limited to, nurse educators, RN director of risk management or quality, RN director of nursing informatics, infection preventionists, and wound ostomy nurses.

The title AVP reflects the function of the role for the purpose of documentation submission. It is understood that registered nurses who function in an AVP role in the organization may not be assigned the title AVP.

certification
"A process by which a state regulatory body or nongovernmental agency or association certifies that an individual licensed to practice a profession has met certain predetermined standards specified by that profession for specialty practice. Its purpose is to assure various publics that an individual has mastered a body of knowledge and acquired skills in a particular specialty" (American Nurses Association 1979, 67).

change
"To undergo transformation, transition, or substitution: winter changed to spring" (Merriam-Webster 2014).

clinical nurse
The registered nurse who spends the majority (≥51%) of his or her time providing direct patient care.

complaint
A written statement expressing dissatisfaction with, for example, service, practice, or professionalism. In contrast, a grievance is a formal complaint filed for resolution with a grievance system or process.

director

Nurses with line authority over multiple units that have RNs working who deliver nursing care in an inpatient or ambulatory care setting and are positioned on the organizational chart between the nurse manager and the chief nursing officer. This may include registered nurses who may broadly influence or impact the clinical practice of nurses in the organization. If these nurses are referenced as a director in the organization's Magnet® application, they must meet the educational criteria (bachelor's in nursing or higher) and report directly or indirectly to the CNO. Examples may include directors responsible for (but are not limited to), nurse educators, RN director of risk management or quality, RN director of nursing informatics, infection preventionists, and wound ostomy nurses.

The title director reflects the function of the role for the purpose of documentation submission. It is understood that registered nurses who function in a director role in the organization may not be assigned the title director.

empirical evidence

"Originating in or based on observation or experience" (Merriam-Webster 2014). Knowledge based on empirical evidence is grounded in scientific findings as opposed to personal belief (Polit and Beck 2012, 11).

enculturation

"The process by which an individual learns the traditional content of a culture and assimilates its practices and values" (Merriam-Webster 2014). This includes the process by which the values of Magnet® are disseminated throughout the depth and breadth of a healthcare organization.

error

"The failure of a planned action to be completed as intended" (an error of execution) "or the use of a wrong plan to achieve an aim" (an error of planning)" (Institute of Medicine 2000, 4). It also includes "failure of an unplanned action that should have been completed (omission)" (Institute of Medicine 2004, 330).

innovation
"Innovation is the application of creativity or problem solving that results in a widely adopted strategy, product, or service that meets a need in a new and different way. Innovations are about improvement in quality, cost effectiveness, or efficiency" (Kaya et al 2015, 1674).

mentor
"An experienced nurse who has developed expertise and can be a strong force in shaping a nurse's identity as a professional" (Anthony, 2006, 73). Mentoring can include providing information, advice, support, and ideas. Typically, mentors and mentees have a long-lasting relationship. The terms 'mentor' and 'receptor' are not used interchangeably.

mission
A statement of the good or benefit the healthcare organization intends to contribute, couched in terms of an identified community, a set of services, and a specific level of cost or finance (Griffith and White 2002, 679).

National Labor Relations Board (NLRB)
"Independent agency created by Congress that oversees relations between unions and employers. The board has the power to settle labor disputes and to enforce its judgments in the federal courts" (Friedman 2012).

nurse managers
Registered nurses with the accountability and supervision of all registered nurses and other healthcare providers who deliver nursing care

in an inpatient or ambulatory care setting. The nurse manager is typically responsible for recruitment and retention, performance review, and professional development; is involved in the budget formulation process and quality outcomes; and helps plan for, organize, and lead the delivery of nursing care for a designated patient care area.

The title 'nurse manager' reflects the function of the role for the purpose of documentation submission. It is understood that registered nurses who function in a nurse manager role in the organization may not be assigned the title nurse manager.

nursing practice environment
"The organizational characteristics of a work setting that facilitate or constrain professional nursing practice." It is a complex construct with theoretical foundations in the sociology of organizations, occupations, and work. The nursing professional practice environment reveals an organization's approach to resolving the dilemmas of "how to organize many workers to perform a large-scale task; how to organize professional staff; and how to organize work that is inherently complex and unpredictable" (Lake 2002, 177, 178).

organization
A stand-alone structure or an entity; the terms can be used interchangeably where appropriate or necessary.

outcome
Quantitative and qualitative evidence related to the impact of structure and process on the patient, nursing workforce, organization, and consumer. "These outcomes are dynamic and measurable and may be reported at an individual unit, department, population, or organizational level" (Malloch and Porter-O'Grady 2010, 267). Donabedian defined outcomes as the "changes (desirable or undesirable) in individuals and populations that can be attributed to health care" (Donabedian 2003, p 46). For Magnet® purposes

an outcome is quantitative evidence related to the impact of structure and process (intervention) on the patient, nursing workforce, organization, and consumer. These outcomes are dynamic and measurable.

patient satisfaction

For Magnet® purposes, "patient opinion of the care received during the hospital stay [or in ambulatory/outpatient services] as determined by scaled responses to a uniform series of questions designed to elicit patient views about global aspects of care" (American Nurses Association 1996).

process

The actions involving the delivery of nursing and healthcare services to patients, including practices that are safe and ethical, autonomous, evidence-based, and focused on quality improvement. Donabedian defined process as the activities constituting health care, "including diagnosis, treatment, rehabilitation, prevention, and patient education—usually carried out by professional personnel, but also including other contributions to care, particularly by patients and their families" (Donabedian 2003, 46).

registered nurse (RN)

A nurse in the United States who holds state board licensure as a registered nurse or any new graduate or foreign nurse graduate who is awaiting state board examination results and is employed by a healthcare organization with responsibilities of an RN. In other countries, this individual will have registered with the appropriate regulatory body.

safety

One of nine optional Magnet® categories for patient satisfaction benchmarking (EP20EO and EP21EO). See also patient safety.

sentinel event

"A patient safety event (not primarily related to the natural course of the patient's illness or underlying condition) that reaches a patient and results in any of the following: death; permanent harm; severe temporary harm" (The Joint Commission 2017, PS-3).

Source of Evidence (SOE)

A statement that describes key elements required to be present and fully operational in a healthcare organization in order to achieve Magnet Recognition®. Sources of Evidence are criteria statements that identify objective indicants of how well the expectations for a Magnet® environment have been met. Source of Evidence statements are distinct from the supporting evidence that may be requested to accompany narratives addressing specific SOEs. See also supporting evidence.

structure

The characteristics of the organization and the healthcare system, including leadership, availability of resources, and professional practice models. Donabedian defined structure as the conditions under which care is provided, including material resources, human resources, and organizational characteristics "such as the organization of the medical and nursing staffs, the presence of teaching and research functions, kinds of supervision and performance review, and methods of paying for care" (Donabedian 2003, 46).

succession planning

"A strategic process involving identification, development, and evaluation of intellectual capital, ensuring leadership continuity within an organization" (Titzer and Shirey 2013, 158).

supporting evidence

Auxiliary documentation provided to support and substantiate narratives to address Magnet® SOE criteria statements. Supporting evidence is required for selected SOEs to provide verification that what is stated in the narrative actually exists in the organization. Acceptable evidence includes, but is not limited to, copies of policies and procedures, meeting minutes, various types of correspondence, data, rosters, and screenshots. Testimonial statements and examples are not acceptable as supporting evidence. See also Source of Evidence (SOE).

transformational leadership

Transformational leaders are "those who stimulate and inspire followers to both achieve extraordinary outcomes and, in the process, develop their own leadership capacity. … [They] help followers grow and develop into leaders by responding to individual followers' needs by empowering them and by aligning the objectives and goals of the individual followers, the leader, the group, and the larger organization" (Bass and Riggio 2006, 3). "Transformational leaders do more with colleagues and followers than set up simple exchanges or agreements—they behave in ways to achieve superior results by employing one or more of the four core components of transformational leadership" (5): idealized influence, inspirational motivation, intellectual stimulation, and individualized consideration.

trended data

Refers to data depicting a trend, defined as "the general movement over time of a statistically detectable change; also, a statistical curve reflecting such a change" (Merriam-Webster 2014). For Magnet® purposes, presentations of trended data to address Empirical Outcomes SOEs must include a minimum of one pre-intervention data point and three post-intervention data points, all occurring within the forty-eight months prior to documentation submission.

vision

An expansion of the mission that expresses intentions, philosophy, and organizational self-image (Griffith and White 2002, 684).

References

Agency for Healthcare Research and Quality. 2015. "Strategies for Improving Patient Experience: Service Recovery Programs." In *The CAHPS Ambulatory Care Improvement Guide: Practical Strategies for Improving Patient Experience* (section 6). Rockville, MD: Author. Retrieved from https://www.ahrq.gov/cahps/quality-improvement/improvement-guide/improvement-guide.html.

American Academy of Ambulatory Care Nursing. 2011. *What Is Ambulatory Care Nursing*. Retrieved from https://www.aaacn.org/what-ambulatory-care-nursing.

American Association of Colleges of Nursing. 2006. *AACN Position Statement on Nursing Research*. Washington, DC: Author. Retrieved from http://www.aacn.nche.edu/publications/position/nursing-research.

American Congress of Obstetricians and Gynecologists. 2011. *Cultural Sensitivity and Awareness in the Delivery of Health Care* (committee opinion number 493). Washington, DC: Author. Retrieved from http://www.acog.org/Resources-and-Publications/Committee-Opinions/Committee-on-Health-Care-for-Underserved-Women/Cultural-Sensitivity-and-Awareness-in-the-Delivery-of-Health-Care.

American Hospital Association. 2017. "Fast Facts on US hospitals." Retrieved from http://www.aha.org/research/rc/stat-studies/fast-facts.shtml.

American Nurses Association. 1979. *The Study of Credentialing in Nursing: A New Approach* (vol. 1, Report of the Committee). Kansas City, MO: Author.

———. 1996. *Nursing Quality Indicators: Definitions and Implications*. Washington, DC: Author.

———. 2015a. *Code of Ethics for Nurses with Interpretive Statements*. Silver Spring, MD: Author.

———. 2015b. *Nursing: Scope and Standards of Practice* (3rd ed.). Silver Spring, MD: Author.

———. 2016. *Nursing Administration: Scope and Standards of Practice* (2nd ed.). Silver Spring, MD: Author.

American Nurses Association and National Nursing Staff Development Organization. 2010. *Nursing Professional Development: Scope and Standards of Practice*. Silver Spring, MD: Author.

American Nurses Credentialing Center. 2008. *Magnet Recognition Program®: Application Manual*. Silver Spring, MD: Author.

———. 2013. *2014 Magnet® Application Manual*. Silver Spring, MD: Author.

———. 2016. *Practice Transition Accreditation Program™: 2016 Application Manual*. Silver Spring, MD: Author.

Anthony, M. K. 2006. "Professional Practice and Career Development." In D.L. Huber (ed.), *Leadership and nursing care management* (3rd ed.), 61–81. Philadelphia, PA: Saunders Elsevier.

Bass, B. M., and R. E. Riggio. 2006. *Transformational Leadership* (2nd ed.). Mahwah, NJ: Lawrence Erlbaum Associates, Inc.

Benner, P., C. Tanner, and C. Chesla. 2009. *Expertise in Nursing Practice: Caring, Clinical Judgment, and Ethics* (2nd ed). New York: Springer Publishing.

Burns, L. R., E. H. Bradley, and B. L. Weiner. 2012. *Shortell and Kaluzny's Health Care Management: Organization, Design, and Behavior* (6th ed.). Clifton Park, NY: Delmar Cengage Learning.

Cain, C., and S. Haque. 2008. "Organizational Workflow and its Impact on Work Quality." In R.G. Hughes (ed.), *Patient Safety and Quality: An Evidence-Based Handbook for Nurses* (AHRQ publication no. 08-0043). Rockville, MD: Agency for Healthcare Research and Quality. Retrieved from https://archive.ahrq.gov/professionals/clinicians-providers/resources/nursing/resources/nurseshdbk/index.html.

DePoy, E., and L. Gitlin. 2016. *Introduction to Research: Understanding and Applying Multiple Strategies* (5th ed.). St. Louis, MO: Elsevier.

Donabedian, A. 2003. *An Introduction to Quality Assurance in Health Care.* New York: Oxford University Press.

Farquharson, J. M. 2004. "Liability of the Nurse Manager." In T.D. Aiken, *Legal, Ethical, and Political Issues in Nursing* (2nd ed.), 311–36. Philadelphia, PA: F.A. Davis Company.

Friedman J. P. (ed.). 2012. *Barron's Dictionary of Business and Economic Terms.* 5th ed. Hauppauge, NY: Barron's Educational Series, Inc.

Gardner, D. B. 2005. "Ten Lessons in Collaboration." *Online Journal of Issues in Nursing* 10 (1): 2.

Gourevitch, M. N. 2014. "Population Health and the Academic Medical Center: The Time is Right." *Academic Medicine* 89 (4): 544–49.

Griffith, J. R., and K. R. White. 2002. *The Well-Managed Healthcare Organization*, (5th ed). Chicago: Health Administration Press.

Grossman, S. C., and T. M. Valiga. 2005. *The New Leadership Challenge: Creating the Future of Nursing*, (2nd ed). Philadelphia: F.A. Davis Co.

Helmreich, R. L. 1998. "Error Management as Organisational Strategy." In *Proceedings of the IATA Human Factors Seminar* (1–7). Bangkok, Thailand, April 20–22, 1998. https://www.coursehero.com/file/6242825/10111312400/.

Institute of Medicine. 2000. *To Err is Human: Building a Safety Health System*. Washington, DC: The National Academies Press.

———. 2004. *Patient Safety: Achieving a New Standard for Care*. Washington, DC: The National Academies Press.

———. 2010. *Redesigning Continuing Education in the Health Professions*. Washington, DC: The National Academies Press.

———. 2011. *The Future of Nursing: Leading Change, Advancing Health*. Washington, DC: National Academies Press.

International Council of Nurses. 2002. "Definition of Nursing." Retrieved from http://www.icn.ch/who-we-are/icn-definition-of-nursing/.

The Joint Commission. 2017. "Patient Safety Systems (PS)." In *Comprehensive Accreditation Manual for Hospitals*, PS1–PS50. Oak Brook, IL: Joint Commission Resources. Retrieved from https://www.jointcommission.org/patient_safety_systems_chapter_for_the_hospital_program/.

Kaya, N., N. Turan, and G. O. Aydin. 2015. "A Concept Analysis of Innovation in Nursing." *Procedia—Social and Behavioral Sciences* 195: 1674–78.

Kindig, D., G. Stoddart. 2003. "What Is Population Health?" *American Journal of Public Health*, 93: 380–83.

Lake, E. T. 2002. "Development of the Practice Environment Scale of the Nursing Work Index." *Research in Nursing and Health* 25: 176–88.

Malloch, K., and T. Porter-O'Grady. 2010. *Introduction to Evidence-Based Practice in Nursing and Health Care*. Sudbury, MA: Jones and Bartlett Publishers.

Merriam-Webster. 2014. *Merriam-Webster's Collegiate Dictionary* (11th ed.). Springfield, MA: Merriam-Webster, Inc.

Mosby. 2017. *Mosby's Dictionary of Medicine, Nursing and Health Professions* (10th ed.). St. Louis, MO: Elsevier.

National Advisory Council on Nurse Education and Practice. 2013. *Achieving Health Equity through Nursing Workforce Diversity*. Retrieved from https://www.hrsa.gov/advisorycommittees/bhpradvisory/nacnep/Reports/eleventhreport.pdf.

National Quality Forum. 2012. *Care Coordination Endorsement Maintenance 2012: Phases 1 and 2: Technical Report*. Washington, DC: Author. Retrieved from http://www.qualityforum.org/Publications/2012/10/Care_Coordination_Phases_I_and_II__Technical_Report.aspx.

Newhouse, R., S. Dearholt, S. Poe, L. C. Pugh, and K. White. 2005. *The Johns Hopkins Nursing Evidence-Based Practice Model*. Baltimore, MD: The Johns Hopkins Hospital and Johns Hopkins University School of Nursing.

Polit, D. F., and C. T. Beck. 2012. *Nursing Research: Generating and Assessing Evidence for Nursing Practice* (9th ed.). Philadelphia, PA: Lippincott Williams and Wilkins.

Shortell, S. M., and A. D. Kaluzny. 2006. *Health Care Management: Organization Design and Behavior* (5th ed.). Clifton Park NY: Thomson Delmar Learning.

Titzer, J. L., and M. R. Shirey. 2013. "Nurse Manager Succession Planning: A Concept Analysis." *Nursing Forum* 48 (33): 155–64.

U. S. Department of Health and Human Services Health Resources and Services Administration. 2011. *Quality Improvement: Quality Improvement Methodology Module*. Retrieved from https://www.hrsa.gov/quality/toolbox/methodology/qualityimprovement/index.html.

Vogt, W. P. 2005. *Dictionary of Statistics and Methodology: A Nontechnical Guide for the Social Sciences*, (3rd ed.). Thousand Oaks, CA: Sage Publications.

Weston, M. J. 2008. "Defining Control over Nursing Practice and Autonomy." *Journal of Nursing Administration* 38 (9): 404–8.

Witmer, A., S. D. Seifer, L. Finocchio, J. Leslie, and E. H. O'Neil. 1995. "Community Health Workers: Integral Members of the Health Care Work Force." *American Journal of Public Health* 85 (8), Pt. 1: 1055–58.

World Health Organization. 2010. *Framework for Action on Interprofessional Education and Collaborative Practice*. Geneva, Switzerland: Author. Retrieved from http://www.who.int/hrh/resources/framework_action/en/.